The Mitochondria Diet Cookbook

Energizing Recipes to Boost Cellular Health, Increase Energy, and Improve Longevity

mf

copyright © 2025 Jeffrey Winzant

All rights reserved No part of this book may be reproduced, or stored in a retrieval system, or transmitted in any form or by any means, electronic, mechanical, photocopying, recording, or otherwise, without express written permission of the publisher.

Disclaimer

By reading this disclaimer, you are accepting the terms of the disclaimer in full. If you disagree with this disclaimer, please do not read the guide.

All of the content within this guide is provided for informational and educational purposes only, and should not be accepted as independent medical or other professional advice. The author is not a doctor, physician, nurse, mental health provider, or registered nutritionist/dietician. Therefore, using and reading this guide does not establish any form of a physician-patient relationship.

Always consult with a physician or another qualified health provider with any issues or questions you might have regarding any sort of medical condition. Do not ever disregard any qualified professional medical advice or delay seeking that advice because of anything you have read in this guide. The information in this guide is not intended to be any sort of medical advice and should not be used in lieu of any medical advice by a licensed and qualified medical professional.

The information in this guide has been compiled from a variety of known sources. However, the author cannot attest to or guarantee the accuracy of each source and thus should not be held liable for any errors or omissions.

You acknowledge that the publisher of this guide will not be held liable for any loss or damage of any kind incurred as a result of this guide or the reliance on any information provided within this guide. You acknowledge and agree that you assume all risk and responsibility for any action you undertake in response to the information in this guide.

Using this guide does not guarantee any particular result (e.g., weight loss or a cure). By reading this guide, you acknowledge that there are no guarantees to any specific outcome or results you can expect.

All product names, diet plans, or names used in this guide are for identification purposes only and are the property of their respective owners. The use of these names does not imply endorsement. All other trademarks cited herein are the property of their respective owners.

Where applicable, this guide is not intended to be a substitute for the original work of this diet plan and is, at most, a supplement to the original work for this diet plan and never a direct substitute. This guide is a personal expression of the facts of that diet plan.

Where applicable, persons shown in the cover images are stock photography models and the publisher has obtained the rights to use the images through license agreements with third-party stock image companies.

Table of Contents

Introduction	9
The Science of Mitochondria and Diet	11
What Is the Mitochondria Diet?	11
Why Mitochondrial Health Is Key to Energy and Longevity	12
Understanding Mitochondria: Your Body's Powerhouse	13
The Link Between Diet and Cellular Energy	14
Getting Started with the Mitochondria Diet	18
How to Build a Mito-Friendly Pantry	18
Essential Nutrients for Mitochondrial Health	20
Meal Planning for Energy and Longevity	23
Energizing Breakfasts to Start Your Day Right	26
Avocado Spinach Energy Smoothie	27
Omega-Rich Chia and Flax Pudding	28
Protein-Packed Veggie Omelets	29
Golden Turmeric Coconut Latte	30
Sweet Potato Breakfast Hash	31
Matcha Energy Bowl	32
Greek Yogurt Berry Parfait	33
Almond Butter and Banana Toast	34
Berry and Spinach Smoothie Bowl	35
Turmeric Sweet Potato Pancakes	36
Power Lunches for Sustained Energy	38
Superfood Quinoa Salad with Lemon-Tahini Dressing	39
Mitochondria-Boosting Chicken and Avocado Bowl	41
Mediterranean Lentil Soup with Olive Oil	42
Grilled Salmon Salad with Anti-Inflammatory Herbs	43
Zucchini Noodles with Pesto and Grilled Chicken	44
Sweet Potato and Black Bean Wrap	45
Broccoli and Cauliflower Power Bowl	46

Wild Rice and Veggie Stir-Fry	47
Spinach and Goat Cheese Stuffed Portobellos	48
Baked Cod with Turmeric and Veggies	49
Dinners that Recharge Your Body	**50**
Herb-Crusted Wild Salmon with Asparagus	51
Grass-Fed Beef Stir-Fry with Ginger and Garlic	52
Baked Cod with Sweet Potato Mash	53
Zucchini Noodles with Creamy Walnut Pesto	54
Lemon Herb Grilled Chicken with Roasted Vegetables	55
Shrimp and Cauliflower Rice Stir-Fry	56
Mediterranean Stuffed Bell Peppers	57
Spaghetti Squash with Turkey Marinara	58
Turmeric Lentil Stew	59
Asian-Inspired Sesame Chicken Lettuce Wraps	60
Snacks and Small Bites for Quick Energy Boosts	**61**
Dark Chocolate Almond Clusters	62
Coconut Matcha Energy Bites	63
Spiced Roasted Chickpeas	64
Greek Yogurt with Blueberries and Honey	65
Avocado and Cucumber Bites	66
Turmeric Spiced Nuts	67
Carrot and Hummus Snack Cups	68
Apple Slices with Almond Butter	69
Hard-Boiled Eggs with Spinach Wrap	70
Cashew Date Bliss Bars	71
Drinks to Support Mitochondrial Health	**72**
Lemon Ginger Detox Tea	73
Green Tea Antioxidant Smoothie	74
Collagen-Boosted Bone Broth	75
Mint and Cucumber Infused Water	76
Turmeric Golden Milk	77

Berry Hibiscus Iced Tea	78
Avocado Lime Smoothie	79
Ginger Beet Juice	80
Almond Chai Latte	81
Spirulina Green Superdrink	82
Sweet Treats That Heal and Nourish	**83**
Dark Chocolate Avocado Mousse	84
Almond Flour Cookies with Cinnamon	85
Baked Pears with Walnut Crumble	86
Coconut Milk Raspberry Ice Cream	87
Cashew Date Energy Bars	88
Sweet Potato Brownies	89
Chia Seed Pudding with Mango	90
Dark Chocolate Dipped Strawberries	91
Banana Nice Cream	92
Pumpkin Spice Bites	93
Meal Plans and Shopping Lists	**94**
7-Day Energy-Boosting Meal Plan	94
Customizing Meal Plans for Your Goals	100
Long-Term Strategies for Energy and Longevity	**106**
How to Incorporate These Recipes into Your Routine	106
Avoiding Burnout: Sustainable Diet Tips	109
Lifestyle Habits to Complement the Mitochondria Diet	110
Conclusion	**115**
FAQs	**118**
References and Helpful Links	**121**

Introduction

Mitochondrial health holds the secret to boundless energy and vitality. These tiny powerhouses within each cell drive nearly every process in the body, from fueling physical activity to sharpening mental clarity, all while playing a critical role in slowing the effects of aging. The often-overlooked connection between what goes on a plate and how efficiently the body generates energy is the foundation of the Mitochondrial Recipe Guides.

Packed with nutrient-dense recipes and practical insights, these guides transform everyday ingredients into powerful tools for optimizing health. With the right balance of antioxidants, healthy fats, and essential nutrients, meals become more than just sustenance—they become a direct route to improving cellular function. Every dish is crafted with care to support mitochondrial performance, reduce oxidative stress, and enhance overall well-being.

In this guide, we will talk about the following;

- The Science of Mitochondria and Diet
- Getting Started with the Mitochondria Diet

- Energizing Breakfasts to Start Your Day Right
- Power Lunches for Sustained Energy
- Snacks and Small Bites for Quick Energy Boosts
- Drinks to Support Mitochondrial Health
- Sweet Treats That Heal and Nourish
- Meal Plans and Shopping Lists
- Long-Term Strategies for Energy and Longevity

Each chapter is designed to inspire, offering breakfasts that set the tone for energetic days, lunches that sustain productivity, and dinners that nourish both body and mind. From simple snacks to indulgent desserts, the recipes seamlessly blend flavor with function, proving that eating for health doesn't mean sacrificing enjoyment.

Keep reading to learn more about how the Mitochondria Diet can help you achieve optimal health and vitality. By the end of this guide, you will have all the tools and knowledge necessary to start incorporating this powerful diet into your daily life. You'll also find tips on how to maintain a balanced approach and make sustainable changes for long-lasting results.

The Science of Mitochondria and Diet

Mitochondria are often referred to as the "powerhouses of the cell." These microscopic structures play a crucial role in energy production, cellular function, and overall health. The foods we consume directly affect mitochondrial performance, and understanding the connection between diet and mitochondria opens up new pathways to improve energy levels, longevity, and well-being.

This chapter explores the fascinating relationship between mitochondria and diet, providing practical guidance for optimizing your health.

What Is the Mitochondria Diet?

The Mitochondria Diet is a nutritional approach aimed at supporting mitochondrial health. The concept revolves around eating foods that promote optimal mitochondrial function while avoiding those that lead to stress, damage, or inefficiency within the mitochondria. This diet isn't about strict calorie counting or adhering to a single fad; instead, it emphasizes balance, nutrient density, and anti-inflammatory foods.

The goal of the Mitochondria Diet is to improve energy production at the cellular level. By fueling the mitochondria with the right nutrients, the body can efficiently convert food into energy, enhance physical and mental performance, and reduce the risk of chronic diseases. The diet focuses on whole, unprocessed foods rich in antioxidants, healthy fats, and essential vitamins while eliminating harmful substances that hinder mitochondrial efficiency.

Why Mitochondrial Health Is Key to Energy and Longevity

Mitochondria are responsible for generating adenosine triphosphate (ATP), the molecule that provides energy for nearly every function in your body. From your brain's activities to muscle contractions, your cells rely on ATP to function properly. The more efficiently your mitochondria work, the better your energy levels and bodily processes will be.

However, mitochondria do much more than produce energy. They regulate cell death, affect immune responses, and play a pivotal role in aging. Poor mitochondrial function has been linked to fatigue, neurodegenerative diseases, cardiovascular problems, and accelerated aging. Supporting your mitochondria ensures that your cells operate efficiently, protecting your body from chronic illnesses and promoting longevity.

Mitochondrial health begins to decline as we age, but diet and lifestyle choices can significantly slow this process. By prioritizing nutrients that bolster mitochondrial function, you can sustain higher energy levels and potentially extend your lifespan.

Understanding Mitochondria: Your Body's Powerhouse

Mitochondria are small, bean-shaped organelles found in nearly every cell of your body, with the exception of red blood cells. Each cell contains hundreds, sometimes thousands, of mitochondria, depending on its energy demands. For example, muscle cells and brain cells have more mitochondria because they require more power to perform their functions.

Mitochondria perform oxidative phosphorylation, a process that converts nutrients into ATP. This process involves oxygen, various enzymes, and the breakdown of carbohydrates, fats, and proteins. However, this energy production is not without cost. It generates free radicals as byproducts, which, if left unchecked, can damage cells. This is where antioxidants, supplied through diet, become essential in neutralizing free radicals and preventing oxidative stress.

Aside from energy production, mitochondria also regulate calcium levels in cells, contribute to immune defense, and influence hormone production, including cortisol and estrogen. Their multifaceted role makes them indispensable for proper physiological function.

The Link Between Diet and Cellular Energy

Mitochondria require a steady supply of certain nutrients to fuel ATP production and maintain their health. Nutrients like Coenzyme Q10, B vitamins, magnesium, and fatty acids are indispensable for metabolic processes. An imbalanced or nutrient-poor diet can lead to sluggish energy production, increased oxidative stress, and mitochondrial dysfunction.

For instance, diets high in refined sugars and trans fats deprive mitochondria of quality fuel and promote inflammation, leading to impaired energy metabolism. Meanwhile, a nutrient-rich diet enhances mitochondrial biogenesis—the creation of new mitochondria—ensuring sustained cellular vitality.

Understanding this connection empowers you to make food choices that directly boost your cellular energy. Eating for your mitochondria helps increase stamina, mental clarity, and overall vitality.

Foods to Boost Mitochondria Function

Choosing the right foods can strengthen and protect your mitochondria. Incorporate these nutrient-rich options into your diet to optimize energy and promote healthy aging:

1. *Leafy Greens:* Spinach, kale, and Swiss chard are rich in magnesium and B vitamins, essential for energy metabolism.
2. *Fatty Fish:* Salmon, mackerel, and sardines supply omega-3 fatty acids, which reduce inflammation and maintain mitochondrial membranes.
3. *Nuts and Seeds:* Almonds, walnuts, chia seeds, and flaxseeds are excellent sources of magnesium and healthy fats to support ATP production.
4. *Berries:* Blueberries, raspberries, and strawberries are packed with antioxidants like anthocyanins, which protect mitochondria from oxidative damage.
5. *Avocados:* This superfood provides healthy monounsaturated fats and potassium to enhance mitochondrial efficiency.
6. *Eggs:* High in protein and B vitamins, eggs support the enzymatic processes involved in energy production.
7. *Dark Chocolate:* Rich in polyphenols, dark chocolate (with 70% cocoa or higher) improves oxygen delivery to mitochondria and supports their function.

8. ***Green Tea:*** Loaded with catechins, green tea stimulates mitochondrial activity and reduces free radical damage.

These foods not only optimize energy but also lower your risk of developing chronic conditions linked to mitochondrial decline.

Foods to Avoid for Better Longevity

Just as certain foods bolster mitochondrial health, others can harm it. To protect your mitochondria and improve longevity, avoid the following:

1. ***Refined Sugars:*** Foods high in added sugars spike insulin levels and lead to inflammation, taxing your mitochondria.
2. ***Trans Fats:*** Found in processed snacks, fried foods, and some margarine, trans fats damage cell membranes and disrupt mitochondrial function.
3. ***Processed Grains:*** White bread, pasta, and pastries are low in nutrients and can cause blood sugar spikes, impairing cellular energy production.
4. ***Alcohol:*** Excessive alcohol consumption creates oxidative stress, depleting antioxidants and harming mitochondria.
5. ***Artificial Sweeteners:*** While marketed as healthier options, some artificial sweeteners may interfere with mitochondrial respiration and energy production.

6. ***Highly Processed Foods:*** These often contain preservatives and additives that contribute to inflammation and oxidative stress.

By reducing or eliminating these from your diet, you provide your mitochondria with a healthier environment in which to thrive.

Your mitochondria are at the heart of your body's energy system, influencing everything from your daily vitality to your long-term health. The Mitochondria Diet focuses on supporting these cellular powerhouses through thoughtful, nutrient-dense eating habits. By prioritizing foods that boost mitochondrial function and avoiding those that harm it, you can unlock the potential for greater energy, improved mental and physical performance, and a longer, healthier life.

Getting Started with the Mitochondria Diet

The Mitochondria Diet isn't just a food trend—it's a lifestyle designed to support your cellular energy systems for optimal health. But as with starting any new habit, preparation is key. This chapter will guide you step-by-step on how to create an environment in your kitchen that sets you up for success.

From reorganizing your pantry, understanding essential nutrients, and cooking with intention to crafting meal plans that truly energize, we'll cover everything you need to know to get started.

How to Build a Mito-Friendly Pantry

A well-stocked pantry is the foundation of any diet, and the Mitochondria Diet is no exception. The right ingredients can make it easier to prepare meals that enhance mitochondrial function. Here's how to craft the perfect mito-friendly pantry:

1. *Focus on Whole Foods:* Ditch heavily processed items and stock up on natural, whole foods. Items like whole grains, nuts, seeds, and dried legumes are

versatile staples rich in nutrients and free from additives that might impair mitochondrial efficiency.

2. ***Healthy Fats are Key:*** Swap inflammatory oils (like soybean or vegetable oil) for healthy fats such as extra virgin olive oil, avocado oil, and coconut oil. These fats support mitochondrial membranes and reduce oxidative stress.

3. ***Stock Up on Spices and Herbs:*** Spices like turmeric, cinnamon, ginger, and rosemary contain antioxidants that combat oxidative damage. Keep these stocked to flavor your meals and provide mitochondrial support.

4. ***Choose Low-Glycemic, Nutrient-Dense Carbohydrates:*** Replace white rice, pastas, and refined flours with alternatives such as quinoa, farro, sweet potatoes, and rolled oats.

5. ***Have Protein Power on Hand:*** Incorporate lean protein sources into your pantry. Canned wild-caught salmon, sardines, and organic, grass-fed jerky are high-quality options for convenient meals. For plant-based eaters, consider lentils, chickpeas, and high-protein grains.

6. ***Limit Sugary and Artificial Sweetened Foods:*** Sugary snacks and artificially sweetened products can impair mitochondrial function. Instead, store natural sweeteners like raw honey or dates for occasional use.

A Sample Mito Pantry

- **Oils:** Extra virgin olive oil, ghee, avocado oil
- **Proteins:** Canned tuna, lentils, almonds, eggs
- **Spices:** Turmeric, paprika, cayenne, black pepper, basil
- **Carbs:** Quinoa, sweet potatoes, steel-cut oats
- **Snacks:** Dark chocolate (70% or higher), raw nuts, dried seaweed
- **Drinks:** Green tea, herbal teas

By being mindful of what you keep in your pantry, you'll set yourself up for easy and consistent adherence to the Mitochondria Diet.

Essential Nutrients for Mitochondrial Health

Mitochondria depend on specific nutrients to function optimally. Incorporating these into your diet ensures that your cells have everything they need to produce energy efficiently and fight off damage. Here are the key nutrients, their functions, and where to find them:

1. **Coenzyme Q10 (CoQ10)**
    - Function: Essential for ATP production and reducing oxidative stress.
    - Sources: Fatty fish (mackerel, trout), organ meats (liver), and spinach.
2. **Magnesium**
    - Function: Facilitates over 300 enzymatic reactions, including those involved in energy creation.

- Sources: Pumpkin seeds, almonds, dark leafy greens, and avocados.

3. **B Vitamins (B1, B2, B3, B5)**
   - Function: Play a key role in converting carbohydrates, proteins, and fats into energy.
   - Sources: Eggs, whole grains, meat, and fortified cereals.

4. **Omega-3 Fatty Acids**
   - Function: Support mitochondrial membranes and reduce inflammation.
   - Sources: Fatty fish, flaxseeds, chia seeds, and walnuts.

5. **Antioxidants (Vitamin C, Vitamin E, Polyphenols)**
   - Function: Neutralize free radicals generated during energy production.
   - Sources: Citrus fruits, nuts, dark chocolate, and berries.

6. **Iron**
   - Function: Essential for oxygen transport and energy production in mitochondria.
   - Sources: Red meat (grass-fed), lentils, and tofu.

7. **L-Carnitine**
   - Function: Transports fatty acids into mitochondria for energy production.
   - Sources: Beef, chicken, and asparagus.

Regularly consuming these crucial nutrients will help you feel more energized and protect your cells from premature aging.

Cooking Tips to Maximize Nutritional Value

How you prepare your food is just as important as the ingredients you choose. Improper cooking can destroy delicate nutrients or create harmful byproducts, so focus on methods that maximize the nutritional value of your meals.

1. ***Favor Gentle Cooking Techniques:*** Methods like steaming, slow-roasting, and sautéing preserve nutrients better than high-heat frying or boiling. For example, steaming broccoli helps retain its vitamin C content compared to boiling it.
2. ***Minimize Overcooking:*** Overcooking food can destroy heat-sensitive compounds, such as antioxidants. Cook food just until done to retain its nutrient density.
3. ***Pair Nutrients for Synergy:*** Combine foods that enhance nutrient absorption. For example, pair leafy greens with healthy fats like olive oil to boost the absorption of fat-soluble vitamins like A, D, E, and K.
4. ***Cut Back on Processed Oils:*** Fats from seed oils break down and release harmful compounds at high temperatures. Stick to stable fats like coconut oil when cooking at high heat.
5. ***Don't Fear Spices:*** Add herbs and spices generously not only for flavor but also for an antioxidant boost. Spices like turmeric are more bioavailable when combined with black pepper and fat sources.

6. *Save the Water:* When boiling vegetables, use the leftover water as broth in soups or sauces to recover water-soluble nutrients that leach into the liquid.

By adopting nutritious cooking habits, you'll enjoy meals that are both delicious and mito-friendly.

Meal Planning for Energy and Longevity

To truly integrate the Mitochondria Diet into your life, planning ahead is essential. Thoughtful meal planning helps reduce stress, save time, and ensure you're consistently providing your body with the nutrients it needs. Here's how to create a weekly plan:

1. *Start with a Balanced Template:* Aim to include a protein, healthy fat, and nutrient-dense carbohydrate with each meal. For example, roasted salmon (protein), avocado (fat), and roasted sweet potatoes (carb) make a simple, balanced dinner.
2. *Batch Cook for Convenience:* Save time during the week by preparing staples in advance. Roast a variety of vegetables like sweet potatoes, broccoli, and zucchini, cook a big batch of quinoa or brown rice, and grill chicken or tofu in bulk. These ready-to-go ingredients make it easy to throw together quick, healthy meals when you're busy.
3. *Snack Smarter:* Avoid reaching for processed snacks by keeping mito-friendly options on hand. A handful

of almonds, walnuts, or trail mix can provide a quick energy boost, while boiled eggs or slices of avocado are great for satisfying hunger while keeping your energy steady.
4. **Prep Ahead:** Simplify your weeknight cooking by doing prep work in advance. Wash and chop vegetables like carrots, peppers, or broccoli and store them in airtight containers. Marinate proteins overnight with your favorite seasonings to enhance flavor and speed up cooking the next day.
5. **Plan for Variety:** Keep your meals interesting and nutritionally balanced by rotating your ingredients. For example, swap out salmon for cod or chicken for turkey to diversify your protein sources. Similarly, alternate greens like kale, spinach, and arugula to ensure you're getting a mix of nutrients and flavors throughout the week.

Sample Daily Mito-Optimized Menu

- **Breakfast:** Scrambled eggs with spinach and avocado, served with a cup of green tea.
- **Snack:** A handful of walnuts and a piece of dark chocolate.
- **Lunch:** Grilled chicken breast over a quinoa salad with arugula and olive oil.
- **Snack:** Celery sticks with almond butter.

- ***Dinner:*** Baked salmon with turmeric-seasoned roasted sweet potatoes and sautéed broccoli.

Planning your meals ahead ensures your body stays fueled and your mitochondria remain nourished throughout the day.

Getting started with the Mitochondria Diet is about creating a sustainable lifestyle that prioritizes mitochondrial health. By organizing your pantry with thoughtful ingredients, focusing on essential nutrients, cooking with care, and planning energizing meals, you can lay a strong foundation for long-term success.

Energizing Breakfasts to Start Your Day Right

Breakfast can set the tone for your entire day. Starting with the right foods gives your body the fuel it needs for sustained energy, mental focus, and cellular health. With the Mitochondria Diet, breakfasts aren't just about quick grabs—they're carefully crafted to support mitochondrial function with nutrients like healthy fats, proteins, and antioxidants.

This chapter brings you ten energizing, delicious, and easy-to-prepare recipes to start every morning on the right note.

Avocado Spinach Energy Smoothie

Ingredients:

- ½ avocado
- 1 cup fresh spinach
- 1 frozen banana
- 1 tablespoon almond butter
- 1 tablespoon chia seeds
- 1 cup unsweetened almond milk (or your preferred plant-based milk)
- ½ teaspoon ground cinnamon (optional)

Instructions:

1. In a blender, combine all ingredients and blend until smooth.
2. Pour into a glass and enjoy immediately.

Omega-Rich Chia and Flax Pudding

Ingredients:

- 3 tablespoons chia seeds
- 1 tablespoon ground flaxseeds
- 1 cup unsweetened coconut milk
- ½ teaspoon vanilla extract
- 1 teaspoon raw honey or maple syrup (optional)
- Fresh berries and chopped nuts for topping

Instructions:

1. In a small bowl, mix chia seeds and ground flaxseeds.
2. In a separate mixing bowl, whisk together coconut milk, vanilla extract, and honey or maple syrup (if using).
3. Slowly pour the liquid mixture into the dry ingredients while stirring continuously until well combined.
4. Cover and refrigerate for at least 2 hours or overnight to allow chia seeds to absorb the liquid and create a pudding-like consistency.
5. Serve topped with fresh berries and chopped nuts for added nutrients and flavor.

Protein-Packed Veggie Omelets

Ingredients:

- 3 large eggs
- ¼ cup diced bell peppers
- ¼ cup chopped spinach
- 1 tablespoon diced onion
- 1 tablespoon olive oil
- Sea salt and pepper to taste

Instructions:

1. Whisk eggs in a bowl with a pinch of salt and pepper.
2. Heat olive oil in a non-stick pan over medium heat.
3. Sauté onions, bell peppers, and spinach until soft (about 2–3 minutes).
4. Pour the eggs over the vegetables, tilt the pan to spread evenly, and cook until the eggs are set (about 3–4 minutes). Flip or fold as desired.
5. Serve warm.

Golden Turmeric Coconut Latte

Ingredients:

- 1 cup unsweetened coconut milk
- ½ teaspoon ground turmeric
- ¼ teaspoon ground cinnamon
- ¼ teaspoon vanilla extract
- 1 teaspoon raw honey (optional)
- Pinch of black pepper (to increase turmeric absorption)

Instructions:

1. In a small saucepan, heat coconut milk over medium heat until hot but not boiling.
2. Whisk in ground turmeric, cinnamon, vanilla extract, and honey (if using).
3. Pour into a mug and sprinkle with a pinch of black pepper.
4. Enjoy as a warm and comforting drink or let it cool and serve over ice for a refreshing twist.
5. Add more spices or adjust the sweetness to your liking.

Sweet Potato Breakfast Hash

Ingredients:

- 1 medium sweet potato, diced
- ¼ cup diced onion
- ½ small zucchini, chopped
- 1 tablespoon olive oil
- 1 handful of arugula or spinach
- 1 soft-cooked egg (optional)
- Sea salt and paprika for seasoning

Instructions:

1. Heat olive oil in a pan over medium heat.
2. Add diced sweet potato and cook until slightly soft (about 5 minutes).
3. Add onion and zucchini, season with sea salt and paprika, and continue cooking until vegetables are tender (another 5 minutes).
4. Serve on a bed of arugula or spinach.
5. Top with a soft-cooked egg for added protein.

Matcha Energy Bowl

Ingredients:

- 1 frozen banana
- 1 teaspoon matcha powder
- ½ avocado
- 1 tablespoon almond butter
- 1 cup unsweetened almond milk
- Fresh fruit and granola for garnish

Instructions:

1. In a blender, combine frozen banana, matcha powder, avocado, almond butter, and almond milk.
2. Blend until smooth and creamy.
3. Transfer to a bowl and top with fresh fruit and granola for added texture and flavor.

Enjoy as a nourishing breakfast or energy-boosting snack.

Get creative with toppings such as nuts, seeds, coconut flakes, or drizzled honey for added sweetness.

Greek Yogurt Berry Parfait

Ingredients:

- 1 cup plain Greek yogurt
- ½ cup mixed fresh berries (blueberries, raspberries, strawberries)
- 2 tablespoons granola or chopped nuts
- 1 tablespoon chia seeds

Instructions:

1. In a glass or jar, layer Greek yogurt, berries, granola or nuts, and chia seeds.
2. Repeat layers until ingredients are used up.
3. Top with a sprinkle of chia seeds for added crunch and nutrition.

Enjoy as a satisfying and protein-packed breakfast or snack.

This parfait can also be made the night before for an easy grab-and-go breakfast option.

Experiment with different fruits and toppings to create your own unique parfait combinations.

Almond Butter and Banana Toast

Ingredients:

- 1 slice of sprouted whole-grain bread
- 1 tablespoon almond butter
- ½ banana, sliced
- Pinch of cinnamon

Instructions:

1. Toast the slice of bread until golden brown.
2. Spread almond butter on top of the toast.
3. Top with sliced banana and a pinch of cinnamon for added flavor.

This quick and easy breakfast or snack is packed with healthy fats, protein, and carbohydrates for sustained energy throughout the day.

For added crunch, sprinkle some chopped nuts or seeds on top before serving.

Drizzle with honey or maple syrup for a touch of sweetness if desired.

Berry and Spinach Smoothie Bowl

Ingredients:

- 1 cup frozen berries (like blueberries and blackberries)
- 1 cup fresh spinach
- ½ cup coconut water
- 1 tablespoon ground flaxseed
- Nuts, seeds, or coconut flakes for topping

Instructions:

1. In a blender, combine frozen berries, fresh spinach, coconut water, and ground flaxseed.
2. Blend until smooth and creamy.
3. Pour into a bowl and top with your choice of nuts, seeds, or coconut flakes for added flavor and texture.

This smoothie bowl is packed with antioxidants, vitamins, and minerals from the berries and spinach.

Switch up the frozen fruit or add in some protein powder for a customizable option that fits your taste preferences.

Enjoy as a refreshing breakfast or snack any time of day.

Turmeric Sweet Potato Pancakes

Ingredients:

- 1 cup mashed sweet potato
- 2 eggs
- 2 tablespoons coconut flour
- ½ teaspoon turmeric powder
- ½ teaspoon cinnamon
- Coconut oil for cooking

Instructions:

1. Combine mashed sweet potato, eggs, coconut flour, turmeric powder, and cinnamon in a mixing bowl.
2. Mix until well combined.
3. Heat a skillet over medium heat and add a small amount of coconut oil.
4. Scoop batter onto the skillet to form pancakes and cook for 2-3 minutes on each side until golden brown.
5. Serve with your choice of toppings such as fresh fruit, nuts, or maple syrup for added sweetness.

These nutrient-dense pancakes are a delicious and unique twist on traditional breakfast pancakes.

Turmeric is known for its anti-inflammatory properties while sweet potatoes provide essential vitamins and minerals for overall health and wellness.

These pancakes are also gluten-free and dairy-free, making them a great option for those with dietary restrictions.

Make a large batch and freeze for easy breakfasts throughout the week.

Start the day with any of these energizing, mitochondria-supporting breakfasts and feel the difference in your energy and vitality. Whether you're blending a smoothie, cooking up an omelet, or grabbing a quick pudding, these recipes will leave both your body and taste buds satisfied.

Power Lunches for Sustained Energy

Lunch marks the midpoint of your day, a chance to refuel your body and recharge your brain. Choosing thoughtfully crafted power lunches can set you up for sustained energy, sharper focus, and better mitochondrial health.

Each recipe in this chapter is designed with the Mitochondria Diet in mind, featuring nutrient-dense ingredients, healthy fats, quality proteins, and antioxidant-rich elements. Whether you're cooking at home or prepping meals ahead, these recipes will keep your cells—and your taste buds—happy.

Superfood Quinoa Salad with Lemon-Tahini Dressing

Ingredients:

- 1 cup cooked quinoa
- 1 cup chopped kale
- ½ cup shredded carrots
- ½ cup diced cucumber
- ¼ cup pomegranate seeds
- 2 tablespoons pumpkin seeds
- 2 tablespoons olive oil

Lemon-Tahini Dressing:

- 2 tablespoons tahini
- Juice of 1 lemon
- 1 teaspoon honey or maple syrup
- 2 tablespoons water (to thin, if needed)
- Pinch of sea salt

Instructions:

1. Combine cooked quinoa, chopped kale, shredded carrots, diced cucumber, pomegranate seeds, and pumpkin seeds in a mixing bowl.
2. Drizzle olive oil over the ingredients and mix well.
3. In a separate small bowl, whisk together tahini, lemon juice, honey or maple syrup, water (to thin), and a pinch of sea salt to create the dressing.

4. Pour dressing over the quinoa salad and mix until evenly coated.
5. Serve immediately or store in an airtight container for up to three days.

Mitochondria-Boosting Chicken and Avocado Bowl

Ingredients:

- 1 grilled chicken breast, sliced
- 1 cup cooked brown rice
- ½ avocado, sliced
- ½ cup sautéed spinach
- 1 tablespoon olive oil
- 1 teaspoon lemon juice
- Pinch of sea salt and black pepper

Instructions:

1. Layer cooked brown rice, grilled chicken slices, sautéed spinach, and avocado slices in a bowl.
2. In a separate small bowl, whisk together olive oil, lemon juice, sea salt, and black pepper to create the dressing.
3. Pour dressing over the chicken and avocado bowl.
4. Serve immediately or store in an airtight container for up to three days.

Mediterranean Lentil Soup with Olive Oil

Ingredients:

- 1 cup cooked green or brown lentils
- 1 tablespoon olive oil
- 1 small onion, diced
- 1 carrot, diced
- 1 celery stalk, diced
- 2 garlic cloves, chopped
- 4 cups vegetable broth
- ½ teaspoon cumin
- ½ teaspoon smoked paprika
- Fresh parsley for garnish

Instructions:

1. In a large pot, heat olive oil over medium heat.
2. Add diced onion, carrot, celery, and chopped garlic to the pot and sauté until vegetables are tender.
3. Add cooked lentils, vegetable broth, cumin, and smoked paprika to the pot.
4. Bring soup to a simmer and let cook for about 15 minutes.
5. Serve hot with fresh parsley for garnish.

Store leftovers in an airtight container in the fridge for up to five days or freeze for longer storage.

Grilled Salmon Salad with Anti-Inflammatory Herbs

Ingredients:

- 1 salmon fillet (grilled or baked)
- 2 cups mixed greens (arugula, spinach, kale)
- ½ cup cherry tomatoes, halved
- 1 cucumber, sliced
- 2 tablespoons chopped fresh dill and parsley
- 1 tablespoon olive oil
- Juice of ½ lemon

Instructions:

1. In a large mixing bowl, add mixed greens, cherry tomatoes, and sliced cucumber.
2. Add chopped dill and parsley to the bowl.
3. Drizzle olive oil and lemon juice over the salad.
4. Toss all ingredients together until well combined.
5. Place grilled or baked salmon on top of the salad.
6. Serve immediately or store in an airtight container for up to three days.

Zucchini Noodles with Pesto and Grilled Chicken

Ingredients:

- 2 medium zucchinis, spiralized
- 1 grilled chicken breast, sliced
- 2 tablespoons homemade or store-bought pesto (preferably olive oil-based)
- Pinch of red pepper flakes (optional)

Instructions:

1. In a large skillet, heat olive oil over medium heat.
2. Add spiralized zucchini to the skillet and cook until softened, about 5 minutes.
3. Remove zucchini noodles from the skillet and place in a mixing bowl.
4. Add sliced grilled chicken and pesto to the mixing bowl with zucchini noodles.
5. Toss everything together until well coated with pesto.
6. Sprinkle red pepper flakes on top for an extra kick of flavor (optional).
7. Serve immediately or store in an airtight container for up to three days.

Sweet Potato and Black Bean Wrap

Ingredients:

- 1 large whole-grain wrap
- ½ cup mashed roasted sweet potato
- ½ cup cooked black beans
- 1 tablespoon Greek yogurt or plant-based alternative
- Handful of chopped fresh cilantro

Instructions:

1. Lay the whole-grain wrap on a flat surface.
2. Spread mashed sweet potato evenly over the wrap.
3. Add cooked black beans on top of the sweet potato layer.
4. Drizzle Greek yogurt or plant-based alternative on top of the black beans.
5. Sprinkle fresh cilantro on top of everything.
6. Roll up the wrap tightly, tucking in any loose ends.
7. Wrap in foil or plastic wrap and store in the fridge for up to three days.

Broccoli and Cauliflower Power Bowl

Ingredients:

- 1 cup steamed broccoli florets
- 1 cup roasted cauliflower florets
- 1 tablespoon tahini
- 1 teaspoon lemon juice
- Sprinkle of sesame seeds

Instructions:

1. Mix steamed broccoli and roasted cauliflower together in a bowl.
2. In a separate small bowl, mix together tahini and lemon juice until well combined.
3. Drizzle the tahini-lemon mixture over the vegetables in the bowl.
4. Sprinkle sesame seeds on top for added texture and flavor.
5. Toss everything together until vegetables are evenly coated with dressing.
6. Serve immediately or store in an airtight container for up to three days.

Wild Rice and Veggie Stir-Fry

Ingredients:

- 1 cup cooked wild rice
- 1 cup mixed vegetables (bell peppers, snap peas, mushrooms)
- 1 tablespoon coconut oil
- 1 teaspoon tamari or coconut aminos

Instructions:

1. In a large skillet, heat the coconut oil over medium-high heat.
2. Add in the mixed vegetables and sauté for 3-4 minutes until slightly softened.
3. Add in cooked wild rice and stir to combine with the vegetables.
4. Drizzle tamari or coconut aminos over everything and continue to cook for an additional 2-3 minutes.
5. Remove from heat and serve immediately or store in an airtight container for up to three days.

Spinach and Goat Cheese Stuffed Portobellos

Ingredients:

- 2 large Portobello mushrooms
- 1 cup fresh spinach, chopped
- 2 tablespoons goat cheese
- 1 teaspoon olive oil

Instructions:

1. Set the oven temperature to 375°F.
2. Remove stems and gills from the Portobello mushrooms.
3. In a small pan, heat olive oil over medium-high heat.
4. Add in chopped spinach and sauté for 2-3 minutes until wilted.
5. Fill each mushroom cap with sautéed spinach and top with crumbled goat cheese.
6. Place stuffed mushrooms on a baking sheet and bake for 12-15 minutes or until cheese is melted.
7. Serve as an appetizer or enjoy as a main dish alongside a side salad.

Baked Cod with Turmeric and Veggies

Ingredients:

- 1 cod fillet
- 1 teaspoon turmeric
- 1 cup mixed vegetables (zucchini, cherry tomatoes, red bell peppers)
- 1 tablespoon olive oil
- Pinch of sea salt

Instructions:

1. Set the oven to 375°F to preheat.
2. In a small bowl, mix together turmeric and olive oil.
3. Place cod fillet in a baking dish and coat with the turmeric mixture.
4. Add mixed vegetables to the same baking dish and sprinkle with sea salt.
5. Bake for 12-15 minutes or until fish is fully cooked and vegetables are tender.
6. Serve with rice or quinoa for a complete meal.

Dinners that Recharge Your Body

Dinner is more than just a meal—it's an opportunity to nourish your body and set the stage for restorative sleep and a day ahead filled with energy. The following recipes are carefully crafted to maximize mitochondrial support. Packed with nutrients, rich in flavor, and simple to prepare, these dinners will recharge your body while satisfying your cravings for wholesome, delicious food.

Herb-Crusted Wild Salmon with Asparagus

Ingredients:

- 2 wild-caught salmon fillets
- 1 bunch of asparagus, trimmed
- 2 tbsp Dijon mustard
- 2 cloves garlic, minced
- 1 tbsp olive oil
- 2 tbsp fresh dill, chopped
- 1 tsp lemon zest
- Salt and pepper to taste

Instructions:

1. Heat your oven to 375°F (190°C) and line a baking sheet with parchment paper.
2. Place salmon fillets on the baking sheet. Spread Dijon mustard evenly over the top.
3. Mix garlic, olive oil, dill, lemon zest, salt, and pepper in a small bowl. Sprinkle this mixture over the salmon.
4. Add asparagus to the baking sheet. Drizzle with a bit of olive oil, and season with salt and pepper.
5. Bake for 12–15 minutes, or until the salmon flakes easily with a fork.

Grass-Fed Beef Stir-Fry with Ginger and Garlic

Ingredients:

- 1 lb (450g) grass-fed beef, thinly sliced
- 2 tbsp coconut oil
- 3 cups mixed vegetables (broccoli, bell peppers, snap peas)
- 2 cloves garlic, minced
- 1 tbsp fresh ginger, grated
- 2 tbsp coconut aminos
- 1 tsp sesame oil (optional)

Instructions:

1. Heat coconut oil in a large skillet over medium-high heat. Add beef and cook until browned. Remove and set aside.
2. Add more coconut oil if needed and stir-fry the vegetables for 4–5 minutes.
3. Add garlic and ginger, cooking for another minute.
4. Return beef to the skillet. Add coconut aminos and sesame oil, stirring to coat everything evenly. Serve hot.

Baked Cod with Sweet Potato Mash

Ingredients:

- 2 cod fillets
- 2 medium sweet potatoes, peeled and cubed
- 1 tbsp olive oil
- 1 tsp paprika
- 1 tsp ground turmeric
- Salt and pepper to taste
- 1 tbsp fresh parsley, chopped

Instructions:

1. Set the oven to 375°F (190°C) and allow it to preheat. Lay the cod on a prepared baking tray.
2. Drizzle olive oil over the cod and sprinkle with paprika, turmeric, salt, and pepper. Bake for 10–12 minutes.
3. Boil sweet potatoes in salted water until tender. Mash with a fork or blender and season with salt, olive oil, or a touch of coconut milk for creaminess.
4. Serve baked cod over the sweet potato mash, garnished with parsley.

Zucchini Noodles with Creamy Walnut Pesto

Ingredients:

- 2 medium zucchinis, spiralized
- 1 cup walnuts, soaked in water for 1 hour
- 1/4 cup olive oil
- 1 clove garlic, minced
- 2 tbsp fresh basil, chopped
- 2 tbsp nutritional yeast (optional)
- Salt and pepper to taste

Instructions:

1. Blend walnuts, garlic, olive oil, basil, nutritional yeast, salt, and pepper in a food processor until creamy.
2. Sauté zucchini noodles in a pan over medium heat for 2–3 minutes until softened.
3. Toss zucchini noodles with the pesto and serve warm.

Lemon Herb Grilled Chicken with Roasted Vegetables

Ingredients:

- 2 boneless, skinless chicken breasts
- Juice of 1 lemon
- 2 tbsp olive oil
- 1 tsp fresh rosemary, chopped
- 1 tsp fresh thyme, chopped
- Salt and pepper to taste
- 3 cups mixed vegetables (carrots, zucchini, and bell peppers)

Instructions:

1. Marinate chicken in a mixture of lemon juice, olive oil, rosemary, thyme, salt, and pepper for at least 30 minutes.
2. Grill chicken over medium heat for 6–8 minutes on each side or until cooked through.
3. Roast mixed vegetables in a 400°F (200°C) oven for 20–25 minutes, seasoned with olive oil, salt, and pepper. Serve together.

Shrimp and Cauliflower Rice Stir-Fry

Ingredients:

- 1 lb (450g) shrimp, peeled and deveined
- 2 cups cauliflower rice
- 2 tbsp coconut oil
- 1 clove garlic, minced
- 1 tbsp ginger, grated
- 1 cup mixed veggies (snow peas, carrots, and green beans)
- 2 tbsp coconut aminos

Instructions:

1. Heat coconut oil in a skillet and cook garlic and ginger until fragrant.
2. Add shrimp and cook for 2–3 minutes on each side. Remove and set aside.
3. Add vegetables to the skillet and cook for 4–5 minutes. Stir in cauliflower rice and coconut aminos. Return shrimp, mix well, and serve hot.

Mediterranean Stuffed Bell Peppers

Ingredients:

- 4 bell peppers, halved and deseeded
- 1 cup cooked quinoa
- 1/2 cup cherry tomatoes, diced
- 1/4 cup olives, chopped
- 2 tbsp fresh parsley, chopped
- 1 tbsp olive oil
- Salt and pepper to taste

Instructions:

1. Set the oven to 375°F (190°C) to preheat. Arrange the bell pepper halves in a baking dish.
2. Mix quinoa, tomatoes, olives, parsley, olive oil, salt, and pepper. Fill the bell peppers with the mixture.
3. Bake for 25–30 minutes or until the peppers are tender.

Spaghetti Squash with Turkey Marinara

Ingredients:

- 1 medium spaghetti squash
- 1 lb (450g) ground turkey
- 1 cup marinara sauce (low-sugar, organic)
- 1 clove garlic, minced
- 1 tbsp olive oil

Instructions:

1. Cut the spaghetti squash in half and remove the seeds. Roast at 375°F (190°C) for 35–40 minutes. Use a fork to scrape out the strands.
2. Heat olive oil in a pan, add garlic, and cook turkey until browned. Stir in marinara sauce.
3. Serve turkey marinara over spaghetti squash.

Turmeric Lentil Stew

Ingredients:

- 1 cup red lentils, rinsed
- 4 cups vegetable broth
- 1 can diced tomatoes
- 1 tsp turmeric powder
- 1 clove garlic, minced
- 1 tbsp olive oil

Instructions:

1. Heat olive oil in a pot, then sauté garlic until fragrant. Add turmeric and cook for 30 seconds.
2. Add lentils, broth, and tomatoes. Simmer for 20–25 minutes until lentils are soft.

Asian-Inspired Sesame Chicken Lettuce Wraps

Ingredients:

- 2 cooked chicken breasts, shredded
- 1 head butter lettuce, leaves separated
- 2 tbsp coconut aminos
- 1 tsp sesame oil
- 1 tbsp sesame seeds

Instructions:

1. Mix chicken with coconut aminos, sesame oil, and sesame seeds.
2. Fill lettuce leaves with the mixture and serve as wraps.

These recipes ensure that dinner is not only delicious but also a time to recharge your body with powerful, nutrient-dense foods. Enjoy creating meals that nourish your energy and vitality!

Snacks and Small Bites for Quick Energy Boosts

Snacks often get overlooked, but they play a crucial role in maintaining energy levels and fueling your mitochondria throughout the day. The right snacks can bridge the gap between meals, stabilize blood sugar, and provide a quick burst of essential nutrients to keep you going.

This chapter brings you ten delicious, nutrient-dense, and easy-to-make snack options that align perfectly with the Mitochondria Diet. Each recipe is designed to provide healthy fats, antioxidants, and proteins to support your body at the cellular level.

Dark Chocolate Almond Clusters

Ingredients:

- 1 cup raw almonds
- ½ cup dark chocolate chips (70% cocoa or higher)
- 1 teaspoon coconut oil
- Sprinkle of sea salt

Instructions:

1. Melt dark chocolate chips with coconut oil in a double boiler or microwave in 30-second increments, stirring until smooth.
2. Toss almonds into the melted chocolate, ensuring they're evenly coated.
3. Drop spoonfuls of the mixture onto a parchment-lined baking sheet, sprinkle with sea salt, and refrigerate until set.
4. Store in an airtight container.

Coconut Matcha Energy Bites

Ingredients:

- 1 cup shredded unsweetened coconut
- 2 tablespoons matcha powder
- ¼ cup almond butter
- 2 tablespoons maple syrup
- 2 tablespoons coconut oil

Instructions:

1. In a food processor, combine shredded coconut and matcha powder until well combined.
2. In a small saucepan, heat almond butter, maple syrup, and coconut oil over low heat until melted.
3. Pour mixture into the food processor and pulse until it forms a dough.
4. Roll into bite-sized balls and refrigerate for 30 minutes before eating or storing in an airtight container.

Spiced Roasted Chickpeas

Ingredients:

- 1 can (15 oz) chickpeas, drained and rinsed
- 1 tablespoon olive oil
- 1 teaspoon paprika
- ½ teaspoon cumin
- ¼ teaspoon garlic powder
- Pinch of sea salt

Instructions:

1. Heat the oven to 400°F and let it preheat.
2. Pat chickpeas dry with a paper towel and remove any loose skins.
3. Toss chickpeas with olive oil, paprika, cumin, garlic powder, and sea salt in a bowl until well coated.
4. Spread chickpeas on a parchment-lined baking sheet and bake for 25-30 minutes or until crispy.
5. Let cool before storing in an airtight container. These make for a great crunchy snack or addition to salads and bowls.

Greek Yogurt with Blueberries and Honey

Ingredients:

- 1 cup plain Greek yogurt
- ½ cup fresh blueberries
- 1 teaspoon raw honey

Instructions:

1. Spoon Greek yogurt into a bowl.
2. Top with blueberries and drizzle with honey. Enjoy immediately.

Avocado and Cucumber Bites

Ingredients:

- 1 small cucumber, sliced into rounds
- ½ ripe avocado
- Sea salt and black pepper to taste

Instructions:

1. Top each cucumber round with a small slice of avocado.
2. Sprinkle with sea salt and black pepper to taste.
3. Serve immediately for a refreshing and healthy snack. Can also be topped with your choice of protein, such as smoked salmon or chickpea salad, for added flavor and nutrition.

Turmeric Spiced Nuts

Ingredients:

- 1 cup mixed raw nuts (almonds, cashews, walnuts)
- 1 tablespoon olive oil (or avocado oil)
- ½ teaspoon ground turmeric
- ¼ teaspoon smoked paprika
- Pinch of sea salt

Instructions:

1. Set the oven temperature to 350°F and allow it to preheat.
2. Mix the nuts with olive oil, turmeric, smoked paprika, and sea salt in a bowl. Stir until evenly coated.
3. Spread nuts on a parchment-lined baking sheet and bake for 10-12 minutes or until lightly toasted.
4. Let cool before storing in an airtight container. These make for a great protein-packed snack on the go or added as a topping to salads or yogurt bowls.

Carrot and Hummus Snack Cups

Ingredients:

- 1 cup baby carrots
- ¼ cup hummus (store-bought or homemade)

Instructions:

1. Arrange baby carrots in a small cup or container.
2. Serve with hummus for dipping.

This easy and flavorful snack is perfect for both kids and adults alike and provides a healthy dose of fiber, vitamins, and minerals.

Apple Slices with Almond Butter

Ingredients:

- 1 medium apple, sliced
- 2 tablespoons almond butter
- Instructions:
- Arrange apple slices on a plate.
- Spread or dip slices into almond butter and enjoy.

Hard-Boiled Eggs with Spinach Wrap

Ingredients:

- 2 hard-boiled eggs, peeled and halved
- 1 large spinach or collard green leaf

Instructions:

1. Lay the spinach leaf flat and place the halved eggs in the center.
2. Roll up and secure with a toothpick if needed.

Cashew Date Bliss Bars

Ingredients:

- 1 cup raw cashews
- 1 cup pitted Medjool dates
- 1 tablespoon chia seeds
- ½ teaspoon vanilla extract

Instructions:

1. Blend cashews, dates, chia seeds, and vanilla in a food processor until a sticky dough forms.
2. Press the mixture into a lined baking dish and refrigerate until firm (about 1–2 hours).
3. Cut into bars or squares and store in the fridge.

These easy-to-make snacks prove that healthy eating doesn't have to be complicated. Each one is designed to fuel your body and mind with the nutrients your mitochondria crave. Try them out and find your favorites to keep on hand for busy days—your cells will thank you!

Drinks to Support Mitochondrial Health

Hydration is key to every cellular process, and drinks designed for mitochondria can offer extra benefits. The right beverages provide antioxidants, minerals, and amino acids, while reducing inflammation and oxidative damage.

This chapter shares ten easy, functional drink recipes to fuel your mitochondria. Each combines practicality with science, keeping you refreshed and energized all day.

Lemon Ginger Detox Tea

Ingredients:

- 1 cup hot water
- Juice of ½ lemon
- 1 teaspoon grated fresh ginger
- 1 teaspoon raw honey (optional)

Instructions:

1. Add grated ginger and lemon juice to hot water. Stir well.
2. Steep for 5 minutes, then strain if desired.
3. Sweeten with honey if preferred. Enjoy warm.

Green Tea Antioxidant Smoothie

Ingredients:

- 1 teaspoon matcha powder or 1 green tea bag brewed in ½ cup water
- 1 frozen banana
- ½ cup spinach
- ½ cup unsweetened almond milk
- 1 tablespoon chia seeds

Instructions:

1. Brew green tea according to package instructions. If using matcha powder, dissolve in ½ cup hot water.
2. In a blender, add brewed tea, banana, spinach, almond milk, and chia seeds.
3. Blend until smooth.
4. Pour into a glass and enjoy chilled.

Collagen-Boosted Bone Broth

Ingredients:

- 1 cup warmed bone broth (chicken, beef, or vegetable-based)
- 1 scoop unflavored collagen powder
- Pinch of turmeric (optional)

Instructions:

1. Warm bone broth in a saucepan or microwave.
2. Stir in collagen powder until fully dissolved. Add turmeric for an anti-inflammatory boost.
3. Sip slowly to enjoy its comforting benefits.

Mint and Cucumber Infused Water

Ingredients:

- 4–6 fresh mint leaves
- 6–8 cucumber slices
- 4 cups filtered water

Instructions:

1. Combine all ingredients in a pitcher or large water bottle.
2. Allow the flavors to infuse for at least 30 minutes before drinking.
3. Enjoy this refreshing and hydrating drink throughout the day.

Turmeric Golden Milk

Ingredients:

- 1 cup unsweetened coconut milk
- ½ teaspoon turmeric powder
- ¼ teaspoon cinnamon
- 1 teaspoon raw honey (optional)
- Pinch of black pepper

Instructions:

1. In a small saucepan, heat coconut milk on medium-high until it begins to simmer.
2. Add turmeric, cinnamon, honey (if using), and black pepper. Whisk until all ingredients are fully combined.
3. Reduce heat to low and let the mixture simmer for 5 minutes.
4. Pour into a mug and enjoy this warm, anti-inflammatory drink before bedtime for a restful night's sleep.

Berry Hibiscus Iced Tea

Ingredients:

- 2 hibiscus tea bags
- 1 cup boiling water
- ½ cup mixed berries (blueberries, raspberries, or blackberries)
- 1 teaspoon raw honey (optional)
- Ice cubes

Instructions:

1. Place tea bags in a heat-safe pitcher or large mason jar.
2. Pour boiling water over tea bags and let steep for 5 minutes.
3. Remove tea bags and add mixed berries to the pitcher or jar.
4. Stir in honey, if desired, and add ice cubes to cool down the drink.

Enjoy this refreshing and antioxidant-rich beverage on a hot summer day.

Avocado Lime Smoothie

Ingredients:

- ½ ripe avocado
- Juice of 1 lime
- 1 cup unsweetened almond milk
- 1 tablespoon flaxseeds
- Pinch of sea salt

Instructions:

1. In a blender, combine avocado, lime juice, almond milk, flaxseeds, and sea salt.
2. Blend until smooth and creamy.
3. Pour into a glass and enjoy this nutrient-dense and creamy smoothie as a meal replacement or post-workout snack.

Ginger Beet Juice

Ingredients:

- 1 medium beet, peeled and chopped
- 1 small apple, chopped
- 1-inch piece of ginger, peeled
- Juice of ½ lemon

Instructions:

1. In a juicer, juice beet, apple, and ginger.
2. Stir in lemon juice.
3. Serve immediately and enjoy this tangy and immune-boosting drink.

Almond Chai Latte

Ingredients:

- 1 cup unsweetened almond milk
- 1 chai tea bag
- 1 teaspoon raw honey
- Dash of cinnamon

Instructions:

1. In a small saucepan, heat almond milk over medium-low heat.
2. Add chai tea bag and let steep for 3-5 minutes.
3. Remove tea bag and stir in honey.
4. Pour latte into a mug and sprinkle with cinnamon.

Enjoy this cozy and healthy alternative to traditional coffee shop drinks.

Spirulina Green Superdrink

Ingredients:

- 1 teaspoon spirulina powder
- 1 cup coconut water
- ¼ cup pineapple chunks
- Juice of ½ lime

Instructions:

1. In a blender, combine spirulina powder, coconut water, pineapple chunks, and lime juice.
2. Blend until smooth.
3. Pour into a glass and enjoy this nutrient-dense and energizing drink to start your day off right.

Sweet Treats That Heal and Nourish

Treating yourself doesn't have to mean sacrificing health. Sweet treats can be nourishing when made with nutrient-rich ingredients that support mitochondrial health. This chapter offers decadent, healing desserts with healthy fats, natural sweeteners, and antioxidants—proof you can indulge while fueling your body the right way.

Dark Chocolate Avocado Mousse

Ingredients:

- 2 ripe avocados
- ½ cup unsweetened cocoa powder
- ¼ cup pure maple syrup
- 1 teaspoon vanilla extract
- Pinch of sea salt

Instructions:

1. In a food processor, blend avocados until smooth.
2. Add cocoa powder, maple syrup, vanilla extract, and sea salt.
3. Blend until well combined and creamy.
4. Scoop into serving dishes and refrigerate for at least 30 minutes before serving.
5. Top with your choice of toppings such as chopped nuts or berries for added flavor and texture.

Almond Flour Cookies with Cinnamon

Ingredients:

- 2 cups almond flour
- ¼ cup coconut oil, melted
- ¼ cup honey or maple syrup
- 1 teaspoon cinnamon
- 1 teaspoon vanilla extract
- Pinch of sea salt

Instructions:

1. Set the oven to 350°F (175°C) to warm up and line a baking sheet with parchment paper.
2. In a large bowl, mix together almond flour, melted coconut oil, honey or maple syrup, cinnamon, vanilla extract, and sea salt until well combined.
3. Using a spoon or cookie scoop, form dough into small balls and place on prepared baking sheet.
4. Bake for 12-15 minutes or until edges are golden brown.
5. Let cookies cool for 10 minutes before serving

Baked Pears with Walnut Crumble

Ingredients:

- 2 ripe pears, halved and cored
- ½ cup chopped walnuts
- 2 tablespoons almond flour
- 1 tablespoon coconut oil
- 1 teaspoon cinnamon
- 1 teaspoon honey or maple syrup (optional)

Instructions:

1. Set the oven to 375°F (190°C) to preheat and line a baking dish with parchment paper.
2. Place pear halves in the dish, cut side up.
3. In a small bowl, mix together walnuts, almond flour, coconut oil, cinnamon, and honey or maple syrup (if using).
4. Spoon mixture onto each pear half.
5. Bake for 20 minutes, or until pears are tender and crumble is lightly golden.

Coconut Milk Raspberry Ice Cream

Ingredients:

- 1 can full-fat coconut milk
- 1 cup fresh or frozen raspberries
- ¼ cup maple syrup
- 1 teaspoon vanilla extract

Instructions:

1. Blend all ingredients in a blender until smooth.
2. Pour mixture into an ice cream maker and churn according to manufacturer's instructions.
3. Transfer to a container and freeze for at least 4 hours before serving.

Cashew Date Energy Bars

Ingredients:

- 1 cup raw cashews
- 1 cup Medjool dates, pitted
- 1 tablespoon chia seeds
- ½ teaspoon vanilla extract

Instructions:

1. Blend cashews in a food processor until finely chopped.
2. Add dates, chia seeds, and vanilla extract to the processor and blend until mixture forms into a ball.
3. Press mixture evenly into an 8x8 inch pan lined with parchment paper.
4. Refrigerate for at least 1 hour before cutting into bars.

Sweet Potato Brownies

Ingredients:

- 1 cup mashed cooked sweet potato
- ½ cup almond butter
- ¼ cup cocoa powder
- ¼ cup maple syrup
- 1 teaspoon vanilla extract
- Pinch of sea salt

Instructions:

1. Heat the oven to 350°F and lightly coat a square baking dish with grease.
2. Combine all ingredients in a mixing bowl and mix until smooth.
3. Pour batter into prepared pan and bake for 20–25 minutes.
4. Let cool before slicing into squares.

Chia Seed Pudding with Mango

Ingredients:

- ¼ cup chia seeds
- 1 cup unsweetened almond milk
- 1 teaspoon vanilla extract
- ½ ripe mango, diced

Instructions:

1. Mix chia seeds, almond milk, and vanilla in a jar or bowl.
2. Let sit for at least 30 minutes, stirring occasionally.
3. Top with diced mango before serving.

Dark Chocolate Dipped Strawberries

Ingredients:

- 1 cup dark chocolate chips (70% cocoa or higher)
- 1 teaspoon coconut oil
- 12 fresh strawberries

Instructions:

1. Line a baking sheet with parchment paper.
2. Wash and dry strawberries, leaving stems on for easier dipping.
3. In a double boiler or microwave, melt chocolate chips and coconut oil until smooth.
4. Dip each strawberry in the melted chocolate, coating about ¾ of the berry.
5. Place on parchment paper and refrigerate until chocolate is set.

Banana Nice Cream

Ingredients:

- 2 ripe bananas, sliced and frozen

Instructions:

1. Add frozen banana slices to a food processor or high-speed blender.
2. Blend until smooth and creamy.
3. Serve immediately or freeze for later use.

Pumpkin Spice Bites

Ingredients:

- ½ cup canned pumpkin puree
- 1 cup almond flour
- 2 tablespoons almond butter
- 2 tablespoons maple syrup
- 1 teaspoon pumpkin pie spice

Instructions:

1. Combine pumpkin puree, almond flour, almond butter, maple syrup, and pumpkin pie spice in a mixing bowl.
2. Mix until well combined and forms a dough-like consistency.
3. Roll into bite-sized balls and place on a parchment-lined baking sheet.
4. Optional: Roll the bites in additional almond flour for coating.
5. Refrigerate for at least 30 minutes before serving.

Meal Plans and Shopping Lists

When committing to a lifestyle change, planning is key. A thoughtful meal plan not only simplifies your daily routine but ensures your body gets the nutrients it needs to thrive. This chapter provides a 7-day energy-boosting meal plan, a convenient shopping list, and tips on customizing your meals to fit your unique goals.

7-Day Energy-Boosting Meal Plan

Each day features meals and snacks designed to nurture your mitochondria with nutrient-dense, energy-enhancing ingredients.

Day 1

Breakfast: Avocado Spinach Energy Smoothie

Snack: Coconut Matcha Energy Bites

Lunch: Superfood Quinoa Salad with Lemon-Tahini Dressing

Snack: Turmeric Spiced Nuts

Dinner Grilled Salmon Salad with Anti-Inflammatory Herbs

Day 2

Breakfast: Omega-Rich Chia and Flax Pudding topped with fresh berries

Snack: Spiced Roasted Chickpeas

Lunch: Mitochondria-Boosting Chicken and Avocado Bowl

Snack: Apple Slices with Almond Butter

Dinner: Steamed Broccoli and Lemon-Turmeric Grilled Chicken with a side of roasted sweet potatoes

Day 3

Breakfast: Protein-Packed Veggie Omelets

Snack: Dark Chocolate Almond Clusters

Lunch: Mediterranean Lentil Soup with Olive Oil

Snack: Greek Yogurt with Blueberries and Honey

Dinner: Baked Cod with Tomato and Olive Tapenade, served with sautéed spinach

Day 4

Breakfast: Lemon Ginger Detox Tea with Cashew Date Energy Bars

Snack: Carrot and Hummus Snack Cups

Lunch: Spinach and Turkey Lettuce Wraps with avocado slices

Snack: Chia Seed Pudding with diced mango

Dinner: Herb-Grilled Chicken with Roasted Cauliflower and a fresh cucumber salad

Day 5

Breakfast: Golden Turmeric Coconut Latte with Sweet Potato Brownies

Snack: Roasted Beet Hummus with cucumber slices

Lunch: Collagen-Boosted Bone Broth with a simple green salad

Snack: Hard-Boiled Eggs with Spinach Wrap

Dinner: Grass-Fed Beef Stir-Fry with colorful bell peppers, ginger, and coconut aminos

Day 6

Breakfast: Green Tea Antioxidant Smoothie

Snack: Dark Chocolate Dipped Strawberries

Lunch: Grilled Shrimp with quinoa and sautéed kale

Snack: Mint and Cucumber Infused Water with Pumpkin Spice Bites

Dinner: Lemon and Garlic Roasted Chicken Thighs with steamed asparagus

Day 7

Breakfast: Banana Nice Cream topped with chopped nuts

Snack: Turmeric Golden Milk with Almond Flour Cookies

Lunch: Wild Caught Tuna Salad with olive oil and lemon dressing, served over mixed greens

Snack: Spirulina Green Superdrink

Dinner: Roasted Salmon with zucchini noodles and pesto sauce

Shopping List for Mitochondrial Superfoods

To follow the Mitochondria Diet effectively, stocking up on nutrient-dense ingredients is key. This expanded shopping list not only categorizes the essentials but also explains their health benefits and offers tips on choosing the best quality options.

With these items in your pantry and fridge, you'll be prepared to whip up meals that support mitochondrial health and promote sustained energy.

Produce

- Spinach
- Avocados

- Lemons
- Ginger
- Cucumbers
- Pears
- Sweet potatoes
- Broccoli
- Cauliflower
- Bell peppers (variety)
- Kale
- Zucchini
- Cherry tomatoes
- Mixed greens
- Fresh herbs (mint, parsley, cilantro, basil)
- Blueberries
- Raspberries
- Strawberries
- Apples
- Bananas
- Mango

Proteins

- Eggs
- Chicken breast and thighs (organic or free-range)
- Grass-fed beef
- Wild-caught salmon, shrimp, and cod
- Bone broth
- Wild-caught canned tuna

- Collagen powder

Nuts and Seeds

- Almonds
- Walnuts
- Cashews
- Chia seeds
- Flaxseeds

Pantry Staples

- Dark chocolate chips (70% cocoa or higher)
- Coconut oil
- Olive oil (extra virgin)
- Almond butter
- Coconut milk (full-fat)
- Quinoa
- Lentils
- Canned chickpeas
- Apple cider vinegar
- Coconut aminos
- Maple syrup
- Honey
- Almond flour
- Turmeric powder
- Cinnamon

Other Essentials

- Greek yogurt (unsweetened and full-fat)
- Matcha powder
- Spirulina powder
- Herbal teas (ginger, hibiscus, mint)

Overall, the Mitochondria Diet focuses on whole, unprocessed foods that are rich in antioxidants, healthy fats, and complex carbohydrates. These ingredients provide essential nutrients to support mitochondrial health and promote overall well-being.

Customizing Meal Plans for Your Goals

Your health is unique, and so are your food preferences, dietary needs, and health goals. The beauty of the Mitochondria Diet is its flexibility. It's not a one-size-fits-all plan but a framework you can adapt to your lifestyle, helping you nourish your body while meeting your specific objectives. Here's a more detailed look at how to customize your meal plan effectively.

1. **Weight Management**

    Maintaining or achieving a healthy weight can feel daunting, but small adjustments to your meal plan can make a big difference. The focus here is on mindful eating and balancing portions.

    - ***Portion Control:*** Healthy high-calorie foods like nuts, seeds, and oils should be eaten in small amounts. Measure a tablespoon of almond butter or pre-portion snacks like nuts or energy bites.

- **Eat the Rainbow:** Fill your plate with fiber-rich, low-calorie veggies like spinach, zucchini, broccoli, and cauliflower. Bulk up meals, like a salmon salad, by adding extra spinach or steamed broccoli.
- **Limit Sugars:** Use natural sweeteners like honey or maple syrup sparingly. For example, sweeten dark chocolate avocado mousse with a small amount of maple syrup instead of refined sugar.
- **Snack Smarter:** Choose nutrient-dense snacks like roasted chickpeas or cucumber sticks with hummus. Keep prepped snacks handy to avoid unhealthy choices.

2. **Vegetarian or Vegan Options**

If you prefer plant-based meals, don't worry—you can follow the Mitochondria Diet while avoiding animal products. The key is ensuring adequate protein and nutrient intake from plant-based sources.

- **Protein Swaps:** Replace chicken, fish, and eggs with plant-based proteins like lentils, black beans, tempeh, tofu, or chickpeas. For example, swap grilled salmon salad for a lentil salad with olive oil and lemon dressing.

- ***Broth Alternatives:*** Use vegetable broth with added nutritional yeast, seaweed, or miso paste for an umami-rich flavor instead of bone broth.
- ***Plant-Based Fats:*** Coconut oil, avocado, nuts, seeds, and tahini are great for healthy fats. Drizzle tahini over roasted veggies or add avocado to lettuce wraps.
- ***Snacks and Treats:*** Try vegan snacks like chia pudding with fruit or sweet potato brownies made without eggs.

3. **Food Sensitivities**

Food sensitivities and allergies shouldn't hold you back from enjoying a meal plan that works for you. The Mitochondria Diet is easily adaptable to dietary restrictions with a few careful swaps.

- Dairy-Free Adjustments: Swap Greek yogurt with coconut or almond-milk yogurt. Use coconut yogurt in parfaits or smoothies.
- Gluten-Free Needs: Choose naturally gluten-free grains like quinoa or rice, and check packaged items like lentils for gluten-free labels. Replace wheat flour with almond flour in baking.

- Avoiding Common Allergens: Replace tree nuts like almonds with pumpkin seeds or flaxseeds in recipes. Use sunflower seeds instead of walnuts for granola toppings.

4. **Busy Schedules**

Life can be hectic, but a little planning ahead can make sticking to your meal plan a breeze, even on your busiest days.

- *Batch Cooking:* Set aside time each week to cook staples like soups, stews, or salads that last for multiple meals. Double recipes like Mediterranean Lentil Soup or roasted veggies to have healthy options ready to go.
- *Prep Basics:* Chop veggies, wash greens, and roast nuts in advance. Store them in airtight containers for quick snacks or easy meals. For example, diced cucumbers and carrots pair perfectly with hummus, and roasted cauliflower makes a quick dinner side.
- *Simplify Snacks:* Keep grab-and-go snacks like almond flour cookies, matcha bites, or energy bars stocked. Portion them into small containers or reusable bags for easy lunches, road trips, or travel days.
- *Meal Storage:* Use high-quality, reusable containers to keep meals fresh and organized.

Look for leak-proof lids and compartments for easy storage. Freeze extras like sweet potato brownies or soups for quick, healthy meals later. Label with dates to stay organized.

5. **Elevating Energy Levels**

    If your goal is to feel more energized throughout the day, focus on including key nutrients and hydration strategies that directly support mitochondrial function.

    - ***Boost Mitochondria with Foods:*** Add CoQ10-rich foods like spinach, parsley, and organ meats to your meals, or snack on magnesium-rich nuts and seeds. Try topping a spinach omelette with parsley for an extra boost.
    - ***Choose Complex Carbs:*** Opt for slow-digesting carbs like sweet potatoes or quinoa, paired with healthy fats and protein for lasting energy. For example, pair roasted sweet potatoes with an avocado lime smoothie.
    - ***Stay Hydrated:*** Drink infused water, like mint cucumber or berry hibiscus tea, to keep your cells hydrated. Dehydration drains energy, so aim for 8+ cups daily.
    - ***Supplement Wisely:*** Consider supplements like magnesium (in seeds and spinach), omega-3s (walnuts, flaxseeds), or CoQ10 if needed.

Practical Tips for Flexibility

Your meal plan isn't meant to weigh you down but to inspire consistency. Here are some overarching strategies to personalize the plan according to your lifestyle:

- *Mix and Match:* Don't be afraid to switch meals between days or double up on favorites. Love Monday's avocado spinach smoothie? Have it twice a week!
- *Try New Recipes:* Introduce variety by experimenting with new dishes, herbs, and spices. A familiar meal can feel entirely different when jazzed up with basil pesto or roasted garlic.
- *Take Small Steps:* If preparing all your meals feels overwhelming, start by focusing on small wins, like consistently prepping snacks or cooking dinner three nights a week.

With these tips, you can confidently tailor your meal plan to meet your health goals while keeping it sustainable and enjoyable.

Long-Term Strategies for Energy and Longevity

Creating lasting changes to your health isn't just about short-term fixes—it's about building habits that support your body and mind for the long haul. This chapter focuses on long-term strategies to help you sustain the Mitochondria Diet, maximize your energy, and promote a longer, healthier life.

Whether it's learning how to seamlessly incorporate these recipes into your routine, avoiding burnout, or adopting complementary lifestyle habits, these tips will keep you energized and inspired for years to come.

How to Incorporate These Recipes into Your Routine

Making nutritious meals part of your everyday life can feel overwhelming at first, but with a little planning and creativity, it becomes second nature. Here are some easy ways to integrate the Mitochondria Diet recipes into your routine.

1. **Plan and Prep Ahead**

   Set aside time each week to plan your meals and snacks. Use a 7-day meal plan as a guide and adjust it to fit your schedule, whether it's a hectic workweek or a relaxed weekend. Planning ahead keeps you organized, saves time, and helps you avoid unhealthy last-minute food choices.

   Batch cook recipes like soups, roasted vegetables, or Coconut Matcha Energy Bites so you always have nutritious options ready. Portion meals into containers for grab-and-go convenience, making it easier to stick to your healthy eating goals all week.

2. **Make Breakfast a Priority**

   Starting your day with a nutrient-packed breakfast sets a positive tone for smarter, healthier choices. A balanced breakfast fuels your body and brain, keeping you focused and energized. Try recipes like the Avocado Spinach Energy Smoothie or Chia Seed Pudding for busy mornings.

   The smoothie is full of healthy fats, fiber, and greens—perfect for an energizing start. Chia Seed Pudding is another easy option—mix chia seeds with milk the night before, let it thicken, and top with mango, berries, or nuts in the morning. Quick, delicious, and satisfying until lunch!

3. **Treat Snacks as Mini-Meals**

   Skip the chips and candy—snack smart with nutrient-packed options like Spiced Roasted Chickpeas or Cashew Date Energy Bars. These tasty choices are full of protein, fiber, and healthy fats to keep you full and energized while stabilizing blood sugar levels to avoid energy crashes. Prep them ahead of time to make healthy snacking easy and stick to your health goals.

4. **Rotate Recipes and Experiment**

   Avoid meal fatigue by rotating recipes and trying new ingredients to keep meals fresh and enjoyable. Use seasonal produce for peak flavor and nutrients, or try dishes from different cuisines—like a Mediterranean quinoa salad with olives and feta or a spicy Mexican twist with jalapeños and lime.

   Customize recipes with herbs and spices to match your taste. Add fresh basil for a vibrant kick in your quinoa salad or sprinkle smoked paprika into sweet potato brownies for a rich, smoky flavor.

5. **Incorporate Mitochondria-Supporting Ingredients Daily**

   To keep your energy up and your cells healthy, include mitochondria-boosting foods in every meal. Leafy greens like spinach and kale support cellular health, while healthy fats from avocados, nuts, and olive oil provide essential fuel. Antioxidant-rich berries like blueberries, raspberries, and strawberries protect mitochondria from damage.

It's simple—add spinach to your smoothie, drizzle olive oil on a salad, or top yogurt or oatmeal with blueberries. Small, consistent habits can make a big difference over time. With a little preparation, these recipes can become part of your weekly routine, keeping your energy vibrant and stress low.

Avoiding Burnout: Sustainable Diet Tips

Sticking to a healthy eating routine can be challenging, but here's how you can make it easier and more enjoyable in the long term:

- *Progress Over Perfection:* Small successes matter. Don't stress over occasional indulgences—focus on steady progress. Swap sugary snacks for healthier treats like Dark Chocolate Almond Clusters and celebrate every positive step.
- *Personalize Your Diet:* Experiment and find what works for your body. Whether it's including grains or going low-carb, listen to how your energy and mood respond to different foods.
- *Plan Ahead:* Prep meals and snacks to avoid unhealthy choices when life gets busy. Stock up on

staples and have recipes ready for quick, mitochondria-friendly options.
- ***Take It Slow:*** Introduce changes gradually. Start by upgrading one meal, like switching to a nutrient-packed smoothie for breakfast, then expand to other parts of your diet over time.
- ***Stay Organized:*** Keep your kitchen stocked and tidy. Plan your shopping and save easy, go-to recipes to reduce the stress of daily meal prep.
- ***Celebrate Wins:*** Reflect on the improvements you notice—better energy, mood, or health—and reward yourself for milestones. Treat yourself with non-food items like fitness gear or a relaxing day off.

By taking a flexible, gradual approach and staying organized, you'll build a sustainable, healthy lifestyle without burnout.

Lifestyle Habits to Complement the Mitochondria Diet

While diet plays a pivotal role in mitochondrial health, your overall lifestyle habits are just as important. Supporting your body with the right practices will amplify the benefits of this diet and create a foundation for long-term energy and longevity.

1. **Move with Purpose**

Exercise boosts your mitochondria—the energy factories of your cells—helping them produce more energy over time. Regular activity improves stamina, cell function, and longevity.

Incorporate a mix of aerobic activities like running or cycling to strengthen your heart and strength training to build muscle and boost metabolism. Low-impact exercises like yoga or walking improve flexibility, balance, and recovery. Even a 10-minute walk after meals aids digestion, regulates blood sugar, and boosts energy.

2. **Prioritize Quality Sleep**

Sleep is essential for your body to repair, recharge, and recover from daily stress. It helps maintain health, improve focus, and boost your immune system. Aim for 7–9 hours of quality rest each night to reset.

To improve sleep, create a calming bedtime routine: dim lights an hour before bed, avoid screens to reduce blue light that disrupts melatonin, and try sipping chamomile or mint tea. Relaxation techniques like gentle stretching, meditation, or journaling can also support deeper, more restorative sleep.

3. **Manage Stress Effectively**

Chronic stress can disrupt mitochondrial function, reducing energy production and affecting cellular health. Managing stress is key to maintaining well-being. Practices like mindfulness meditation to clear your mind, deep breathing to trigger relaxation, or a 20-minute walk in nature can lower cortisol and improve mood.

Simple habits like journaling to process emotions or gratitude exercises to focus on positives are also powerful tools. These small, consistent actions can boost both mental and physical resilience.

4. Stay Hydrated

Water is a pillar of cellular health, playing a crucial role in keeping your body functioning at its best. Proper hydration supports your mitochondria, the energy powerhouses of your cells, ensuring they perform optimally throughout the day. Staying hydrated can also improve your focus, energy levels, and even your skin.

To make hydration more enjoyable, try preparing refreshing infused waters like Mint and Cucumber Infused Water or Lemon Ginger Tea. These simple yet flavorful drinks are easy to make and are perfect to sip on throughout the day, keeping you both hydrated and invigorated.

5. Cultivate Gratitude and Joy

A positive mindset can greatly improve your health and longevity. Surround yourself with supportive relationships, whether it's family, friends, or a community that uplifts you.

Take time each day to reflect on what you're thankful for, no matter how small.

Do activities that bring you joy, like a favorite hobby, spending time in nature, or trying something new. Studies show that happiness and social connections reduce stress, boost your immune system, and improve mental and physical well-being.

6. Limit Toxins

Environmental toxins like processed foods, cigarette smoke, heavy metals, and pollutants can harm mitochondria, the energy producers in your cells. These toxins cause oxidative stress, damaging mitochondria and impacting overall health.

To limit exposure, choose organic produce to avoid pesticides, cut back on processed foods, and use natural, eco-friendly cleaning products. Small, consistent changes can protect your mitochondria and support long-term cell health.

7. Stay Consistent

Consistency in diet and lifestyle matters more than chasing perfection. It's not about being perfect every day but about making small, sustainable choices that add up. For example, plan a weekly exercise routine, even just 20 minutes a day, and keep healthy snacks like nuts or fruit handy to avoid less nutritious options.

These small changes will gradually become habits and feel natural, helping you maintain a healthier, balanced lifestyle over time. The Mitochondria Diet then shifts from a short-term goal to a lasting way of life. By fueling your body with nutritious food, prioritizing rest and movement, and staying positive, you're building long-term energy, health, and longevity.

Conclusion

Thank you for taking the time to explore the Mitochondrial Cookbook Recipe Guides. You've taken a meaningful step toward prioritizing not just your overall health but also the foundation of your well-being—your cellular energy system. By reading through this guide, you've equipped yourself with tools, knowledge, and recipes designed to empower your mitochondria, the tiny yet mighty powerhouses of your cells.

The importance of nurturing your mitochondria can't be overstated. They influence so much more than energy production—they are key players in your immune function, metabolism, focus, and even longevity. When you prioritize what fuels these cellular engines through thoughtful nutrition and smart lifestyle choices, you set the stage for sustained vitality and improved quality of life. It's proof that small, consistent actions, like choosing the right foods or prepping nourishing snacks, can have profound long-term effects.

The recipes we've shared were crafted with intention—to balance functionality with flavor, science with convenience. You've seen how you can integrate nutrient-packed dishes into your routine without it feeling overwhelming or restrictive. Eating for your mitochondria doesn't mean giving up joy at mealtime. It means reimagining how food can enhance your health while still indulging your taste buds. Perhaps you now see breakfast as an opportunity to "set the tone" for your day with an Avocado Spinach Energy Smoothie or a Protein-Packed Veggie Omelet. Or maybe you'll elevate snack time with Dark Chocolate Almond Clusters or treat yourself guilt-free to a luscious Dark Chocolate Avocado Mousse. These recipes are proof that caring for your health is not only doable—it's delicious.

Now, here's where you take charge. Remember, you don't have to implement change all at once. Consistency matters more than perfection. Start small—swap one or two meals, carve out time to batch-cook snacks, or simply add a leafy green salad to your lunch routine. Before you know it, your diet will naturally revolve around whole, unprocessed foods that support mitochondrial health.

Your kitchen is your lab, and you are the chef of your own well-being. Don't be afraid to experiment, customize recipes, or even create your own versions of meals using what you've learned. What matters most is that you're taking ownership of this part of your health. Over time, these choices become habits, and those habits build the foundation for longevity and vitality.

Lastly, be patient with yourself. Embarking on a lifestyle rooted in health doesn't mean perfection every day. Life happens, and flexibility is key. Forgive any setbacks and focus on the progress you're making. Celebrate your wins, even the small ones—whether it's swapping processed snacks for something wholesome or discovering a new favorite recipe. These victories all contribute to creating a life that feels truly energized and balanced.

The power is in your hands. Each meal, every mindful choice, brings you closer to a healthier, more vibrant version of yourself. Your mitochondria will thank you with better energy, sharper focus, and a true zest for life. Thank you for joining us on this mission to nourish your cells—and yourself. Here's to your health, your energy, and your bright future.

If you found this guide helpful and would like to explore the mitochondria diet in greater detail, simply scan the QR code to access the companion edition of this guide.

FAQs

Why is mitochondrial health so important for overall well-being?

Mitochondria are the energy powerhouses of your cells, playing a key role in producing the energy your body needs to function. They also influence your immune system, metabolism, and even how you age. When you nurture your mitochondria through thoughtful nutrition and lifestyle choices, you support sustained energy, improved focus, and overall vitality.

How do I get started with the Mitochondrial Cookbook Recipe Guides?

Start small and make gradual changes. Begin by swapping one or two meals a day with the mitochondria-friendly recipes from the guide. For example, try the Avocado Spinach Energy Smoothie for breakfast or the Dark Chocolate Almond Clusters as a healthy snack. Taking it one step at a time ensures the changes feel manageable and sustainable.

Are these recipes time-consuming to prepare?

Not at all! Many recipes in the guide are quick and easy to make, perfect for busy schedules. With a little planning, like batch-cooking snacks or prepping ingredients in advance, you can save time during the week while still enjoying nutrient-packed meals. Even simple dishes, like the Protein-Packed Veggie Omelets, come together in minutes and deliver plenty of flavor and nourishment.

What if I'm not a great cook? Can I still follow these recipes?

Yes, absolutely! The recipes are designed to be approachable for both beginners and experienced cooks. Clear instructions guide you through every step, and the ingredients are simple and easy to find. Remember, your kitchen is your lab—don't be afraid to experiment and customize recipes to suit your tastes.

What should I do if I fall off track?

Don't worry—this is normal! What's important is progress, not perfection. If you have a setback, focus on getting back on course with your next meal or snack. Celebrate the small wins, whether it's choosing a healthier snack or trying a new recipe. Flexibility and self-compassion will keep you motivated over the long term.

How can I make these recipes a regular part of my lifestyle?

Consistency is key. Plan your meals ahead, stock your pantry with essentials, and use the recipes as inspiration for your weekly menu. Batch-cook staples like roasted vegetables or energy bites, so you always have something healthy ready to go. Over time, these choices will naturally become habits that fit into your routine.

Can nourishing my mitochondria really make a noticeable difference in my energy levels?

Absolutely! By prioritizing nutrient-dense foods and eliminating those that harm mitochondrial function, you're giving your cells the tools they need to perform at their best. Many people notice higher energy, mental clarity, and improved focus after incorporating these changes into their diet. Stick with it and give your body the time it needs to reap the rewards.

References and Helpful Links

Juicer, P. (2022, April 6). Recipes to Support Mitochondrial Health - PURE Juicer blog. PURE Juicer Blog. https://blog.purejuicer.com/2021/09/02/five-delicious-juice-recipes-to-boost-mitochondrial-health/

Mitochondria diet. (2025, January 3). Root Functional Medicine. https://rootfunctionalmedicine.com/mitochondria-diet

Wild Nutrition® Ltd. (2024, August 21). 8 Ways to support your mitochondria. https://www.wildnutrition.com/blogs/our-blog/8-ways-to-support-your-mitochondria

Rd, C. S. M. (2024, June 19). What to eat to help you live longer and healthier. Health. https://www.health.com/nutrition/longevity-diet

THE PCCA BLOG | Mitochondrial health: the key to longevity? (2024, September 25). https://www.pccarx.com/Blog/mitochondrial-health-the-key-to-longevity#:~:text=These%20tiny%20organelles%2C%20often%20referred,oxidative%20stress%20and%20accelerated%20aging.

News-Medical. (2024, March 19). Beyond Energy: Mitochondria's role in Diet and health.
https://www.news-medical.net/health/Beyond-Energy-Mitochondrias-Role-in-Diet-and-Health.aspx

IFM Mito Food Plan | Nourishing Meals®. (n.d.).
https://nourishingmeals.com/diet/ifm-mito-food-plan

www.ingramcontent.com/pod-product-compliance
Lightning Source LLC
LaVergne TN
LVHW021224080526
838199LV00089B/5822